Table of Contents

The main symptom of collagenous colitis and lymphocytic colitis is chronic, watery diarrhea, as often as five to 10 watery bowel movements per day. More than half of patients cannot pinpoint when their symptoms began.

The diarrhea is usually accompanied by cramps and abdominal pain. These episodes rarely occur at night. Patients are commonly given an incorrect diagnosis of irritable bowel syndrome. One key difference is that patients with collagenous/lymphocytic colitis tend to be older and do not have a history of alternating constipation and diarrhea.

BREAKFAST

1. Casserole

Prep Time: 20 Minutes

Cook Time: 45 Minutes

Servings: 12

Ingredients

- 4 cups (175g or 6 oz) cubes of crusty bread
- 1 teaspoon olive oil
- 1 pound ground pork sausage, casings removed
- 1 teaspoon dried rosemary or Italian seasoning, optional
- 1/2 medium onion, diced (115g or 3/4 cup)
- 2 garlic cloves, minced
- 2 cups (275g or 9–10 oz) diced bell peppers
- 1 cup (100g or 3 oz) sliced mushrooms
- 1 cup roughly chopped fresh spinach
- 12 large eggs
- 1/4 teaspoon salt

- 1/8 teaspoon freshly ground black pepper

- 2/3 cup (160ml) milk or half-and-half

- 1 cup (100g or 3.5 oz.) shredded cheddar cheese

Optional garnish:

- green onion and/or chopped parsley

Instructions

1. Grease a 9×13-inch or any 3–4-quart oven-safe dish. Arrange bread cubes in an even layer in bottom of pan.

2. Heat olive oil in a large skillet over medium heat. Add sausage and rosemary/Italian seasoning, if using, and break up the sausage into bite-size pieces with a wooden spoon or rubber spatula as it begins to cook. Add the onion, garlic, peppers, mushrooms, and spinach and cook until everything has slightly softened and sausage is mostly cooked through, about 5–6 minutes.

3. Remove sausage and vegetable mixture from heat and spread in an even layer on top of bread.

4. Whisk the eggs, salt, pepper, milk, and cheese together. Evenly pour over sausage/vegetable

mixture. Add another sprinkle of salt and pepper on top.

5. Cover casserole with plastic wrap or aluminum foil and refrigerate for at least 30 minutes and up to 24 hours. (When ready to bake, allow to sit at room temperature for 10–15 minutes as oven preheats.)

6. Preheat the oven to 375°F (191°C). Bake the casserole, uncovered, until the top is golden, edges are crisp, and a toothpick inserted in the center comes out clean, about 40–45 minutes.

7. Cool for 10 minutes, then slice and serve.

8. Leftovers keep well in the refrigerator for up to 5 days. Reheat in the microwave to your liking.

Prep Time: 30 Minutes

Cook Time: 50 Minutes

Servings: 12

Ingredients

- 1 (12-14 ounce) loaf french bread, sourdough bread, or challah
- 8 ounces (224g) block cream cheese, softened to room temperature
- 2 Tablespoons (15g) confectioners' sugar (do not leave out)
- 3 teaspoons (15ml) pure vanilla extract, divided
- 8 large eggs
- 2 and 1/4 cups (540ml) whole milk
- 3/4 teaspoon ground cinnamon
- 2/3 cup (133g) packed light brown sugar

Crumb Topping

- 1/3 cup (69g) packed light brown sugar
- 1/3 cup (41g) all-purpose flour (spoon & leveled)
- 1/2 teaspoon ground cinnamon

- 6 Tablespoons (86g) unsalted butter, cold and cubed

Optional:

- maple syrup and/or confectioners' sugar for topping

Instructions

1. Grease a 9×13 inch or any 3-4 quart oven-safe dish with nonstick spray. Slice then cut the bread into cubes, about 1 inch in size. Spread half of the cubes into the prepared baking pan.
2. Using a handheld or stand mixer fitted with a whisk attachment, beat the room temperature cream cheese on medium-high speed until completely smooth. Beat in the confectioners' sugar and 1/4 teaspoon vanilla extract until combined. Drop random spoonfuls of cream cheese mixture on top of the bread. Layer the remaining bread cubes on top of cream cheese. (I like to make sure some cream cheese is still exposed on top just for looks.) Set aside.
3. Whisk the eggs, milk, cinnamon, brown sugar, and remaining vanilla together until no brown sugar lumps remain. Pour evenly over the bread. Cover the

pan tightly with plastic wrap and refrigerate for at least 3-4 hours and up to 24 hours. Overnight is best.

4. Preheat oven to 350°F (177°C). Remove pan from the refrigerator.

5. Prepare the crumb topping: Whisk the brown sugar, flour, and cinnamon together in a medium bowl. Cut in the cold cubed butter with a pastry blender or two forks. Sprinkle the topping evenly over the soaked bread.

6. Bake uncovered for 45-55 minutes or until golden brown on top. I usually bake it for 45 minutes because I like it softer. Drizzle with optional maple syrup or dust with confectioners' sugar. Serve warm.

7. Cover leftovers tightly and store in the refrigerator for 2-3 days.

Prep Time: 30 Minutes

Cook Time: 50 Minutes

Servings: 12

Ingredients

- 1 (12-14 ounce) loaf french bread, sourdough bread, or challah
- 1 cup (227g) pumpkin puree
- 3/4 cup (150g) packed light or dark brown sugar
- 2 and 1/2 teaspoons store-bought or homemade pumpkin pie spice
- 6 large eggs
- 2 and 1/3 cups (560ml) whole milk
- 2 teaspoons pure vanilla extract

Crumb Topping

- 1/3 cup (69g) packed light brown sugar
- 1/3 cup (41g) all-purpose flour (spoon & leveled)
- 1/2 teaspoon ground cinnamon
- 6 Tablespoons (86g) unsalted butter, cold and cubed
- 3/4 cup (100g) roughly chopped pecans

For serving:

- pure maple syrup

Instructions

1. Slice and cut the bread into 1-inch cubes. Let the cubed bread sit out uncovered for a few hours or up to 1 day. (If you don't have enough time, see Bread note below.)

2. Grease a 9×13 inch (or any 3.5-4 quart) baking dish or spray with nonstick spray. Spread cubes of bread in the dish.

3. Whisk pumpkin, brown sugar, pumpkin pie spice, eggs, milk, and vanilla extract together in a large bowl. Pour evenly over bread.

4. Cover the pan tightly and place in the refrigerator for at least 3 hours and up to 1 day. This gives the bread a chance to soak up the pumpkin custard and is a key step in this recipe.

5. Make and refrigerate the crumb topping too: Mix the brown sugar, flour, and cinnamon together. Add the cold butter and using a pastry cutter or fork, cut butter into the brown sugar mixture until pea-size crumbles form. You can also use your hands to mix it

together. Stir in the pecans. Cover and refrigerate (separately, do not add to soaking casserole) until ready to use in step 7. Can be refrigerated for just 15 minutes or up to 1 day. The colder it is, the less likely it will sink down and get lost in the casserole.

6. Remove casserole the refrigerator and preheat oven to 350°F (177°C).

7. Sprinkle crumb topping evenly over casserole and bake uncovered for 20 minutes, and then cover with aluminum foil and bake for an additional 25-35 minutes or until center appears set and is no longer runny. The total time this casserole takes is 45-55 minutes.

8. Remove from the oven and cool for 5 minutes before serving. Casserole deflates slightly as it cools. Feel free to drizzle maple syrup on top of entire casserole or on individual servings.

9. Cover leftovers tightly and store in the refrigerator for 2-3 days.

Prep Time: 1hrs, 30 Minutes

Cook Time: 55 Minutes

Servings: 10-12

Ingredients

- 8 cups (about a 12 ounce loaf) cubed bread (I recommend big chunks of a crispy baguette or sourdough loaf)
- 8 slices uncooked bacon
- 1/2 cup chopped onion
- 3 garlic cloves, finely minced
- 3 packed cups fresh chopped spinach
- 1 and 1/2 cups shredded parmesan cheese
- 9 large eggs
- 2 cups whole milk
- 1 teaspoon salt
- 1 teaspoon ground mustard
- 1/4 teaspoon fresh ground black pepper

Optional garnish:

- fresh ground black pepper, flaky sea salt, and/or extra parmesan cheese

Instructions

1. Grease a 9×13 inch (or similar size) casserole dish or spray with nonstick spray.
2. Arrange bread in a single layer in the pan, then set pan aside.
3. Cook bacon according to package stovetop directions in a large skillet. Drain all but about 1 Tablespoon grease. (Or drain it all and add 1 Tablespoon olive oil for the next step.) Cool bacon until ready to handle, then chop into bite-size pieces. Sprinkle over bread.
4. Add onion to greased skillet. Cook on medium heat until soft, about 4 minutes. Add garlic and spinach and while stirring occasionally, cook until spinach has wilted, about 2-3 minutes. Remove from heat. Spoon evenly over the bread/bacon, then sprinkle all of the cheese on top.
5. Whisk eggs, milk, salt, ground mustard, and pepper together in a large bowl. Pour evenly over cheese. Cover tightly and refrigerate for 1 hour or overnight (up to 12-16 hours).

6. Remove casserole from the refrigerator and allow to sit out at room temperature for 15 minutes.

7. Preheat the oven to 375°F (191°C).

8. Bake casserole, uncovered, for 20 minutes. Loosely cover with aluminum foil and bake for 30-35 minutes. The casserole is done when browned on the sides and puffy in the center– usually takes 50-55 minutes total.

9. Remove from the oven, sprinkle optional garnish(es) on top if using, and allow to cool for 5 minutes before serving.

10. Cover leftovers tightly and store in the refrigerator for up to 5 days. Reheat in the microwave.

Prep Time: 15 Minutes

Cook Time: 45 Minutes

Servings: 12

Ingredients

- 3 day-old everything bagels, cut into bite-size pieces (about 6 cups)
- 1 bell pepper, chopped
- 3/4 cup quartered cherry tomatoes (or chopped regular tomato)
- 6 slices cooked bacon, chopped
- 9 large eggs
- 1 and 1/2 cups whole milk
- 1 and 1/2 cups shredded cheese
- 1/2 teaspoon ground mustard
- 1/4 teaspoon salt
- 1/8 teaspoon freshly ground black pepper
- 6 ounces block cream cheese, cut into bite-size pieces

Optional for garnish:

- everything bagel seasoning and scallions

Instructions

1. Preheat the oven to 375°F (191°C). Generously grease a 9×13 inch baking pan or similar size (about 3 quart) casserole dish.

2. Layer the bagel pieces, chopped pepper, tomatoes, and bacon into the dish. Whisk the eggs, milk, cheese, ground mustard, salt, and pepper together in a large bowl. Pour evenly over bagel mixture.

3. Top evenly with pieces of cream cheese and sprinkle with everything bagel seasoning, if using.

4. Bake for 40-50 minutes or until center is set and edges are golden brown. Remove from the oven and allow to cool for 10 minutes before topping with scallions (if using), slicing, and serving.

5. Cover leftover casserole tightly and refrigerate for up to 1 week.

Prep Time: 5 Minutes

Cook Time: 35 Minutes

Servings: 9

Ingredients

- 1 and 3/4 cups (420ml) milk
- 2 large eggs
- 1/2 cup (120ml) pure maple syrup
- 1/4 cup (60g) unsalted butter, melted and slightly cooled
- 1/4 cup (60g) unsweetened applesauce or mashed banana
- 3 cups (240g) old-fashioned whole oats
- 1 teaspoon baking powder
- 1 teaspoon ground cinnamon
- 1 teaspoon pure vanilla extract
- 1/4 teaspoon salt
- 1 and 1/2 cups mixed berries, fresh or frozen (do not thaw)

Optional for topping:

- 1/2 cup chopped walnuts or pecans

Instructions

1. Adjust the oven rack to the lower third position and preheat the oven to 350°F (177°C). Spray a 9×9 inch or 11×7 inch baking pan with nonstick spray. Any similar size or shape pan works, though 8×8 inch would be too small. See recipe note for 9×13 inch pan.
2. Whisk all of the ingredients together in 1 large bowl. Pour into prepared baking pan. Top with nuts, if desired. (Or stir into the oatmeal.) Bake for 35 minutes or until the center appears almost set, which gives us a soft oatmeal as pictured above. For drier and more solid baked oatmeal, bake until center has set.
3. Cool for 5 minutes before serving. Spoon or slice and serve with yogurt, if desired. Cover leftovers tightly and refrigerate for up to 1 week.

Prep Time: 8hrs, 15 Minutes

Cook Time: 55 Minutes

Servings: 10-12

Ingredients

- 8–10 cups (12–14 ounces weight) cubed bread (I recommend big chunks of a crispy baguette)
- 1/2 cup diced tomato
- 1/2 cup diced green bell pepper (or any color)
- 2 cups cooked and cubed ham
- 2 cups shredded cheese (I use a mix of gouda and mozzarella)
- 9 large eggs
- 2 cups milk (any kind)
- 1 teaspoon salt
- 1 teaspoon smoked paprika
- 1 teaspoon ground mustard
- 1/4 teaspoon fresh ground black pepper, plus more for topping
- 2 Tablespoons green onion

Instructions

1. Generously grease a 9×13 inch (or similar size) casserole dish or spray with nonstick spray.
2. Layer in the bread, then the peppers, tomatoes, and ham. Sprinkle cheese evenly over top.
3. Whisk the eggs, milk, salt, ground mustard, smoked paprika, and pepper together. Pour evenly over other ingredients in the casserole dish. Top with scallions and a little more pepper, if desired.
4. Cover tightly and refrigerate for 1 hour or overnight (up to 12-16 hours).
5. Remove casserole from the refrigerator and allow to sit out at room temperature for 15 minutes.
6. Preheat the oven to 375°F (191°C).
7. Bake casserole, uncovered, for 30 minutes. Loosely cover with aluminum foil for the remaining 20-30 minutes. Casserole is done with browned on the sides and puffy in the center. Mine usually takes about 55 minutes.
8. Remove from the oven and allow to cool for 5 minutes before serving.
9. Cover leftovers tightly and store in the refrigerator for up to 5 days. Reheat in the microwave.

Prep Time: 20 Minutes

Cook Time: 20 Minutes

Servings: 6

Ingredients

- 6 Tortillas or wraps
- 2 batches Vegan Scrambled Eggs
- 1 tablespoon oil
- ½ red onion diced
- 2-3 cloves garlic minced
- ½ red pepper diced
- ½ green pepper diced
- ½ teaspoon cumin
- ½ cup salsa, store bought or homemade
- ¼ cup green chilies
- 1 (14 oz) can black beans
- Juice of 1 lime
- Salt and pepper to taste
- 1 cup non-dairy cheese optional

Instructions

1. Preheat the oven to 350 degrees F.

2. Begin by making the vegan scrambled eggs. Once done, transfer to a bowl and set aside.

3. In the same skillet, heat 1 tablespoon of coconut oil. Add onions and sauté for 5 minutes, until tender and fragrant. Add garlic and red and green peppers, and continue cooking for another 5-7 minutes until peppers are tender. Add green chiles, cumin, black beans, and lime juice. Cook for about 3 more minutes. Stir in vegan scrambled eggs and remove from heat.

4. Evenly divide the filling between the 6 wraps. Sprinkle with non-dairy cheese and roll up. Place on a baking sheet, seam side down, and bake for 20 minutes.

Prep Time: 40 Minutes

Cook Time: 10 Minutes

Servings: 4

Ingredients

- 2 medium Russet or Yukon Gold potatoes (or sweet potatoes)
- 3 strips bacon
- 1 large bell pepper, chopped (I used 1/2 of a red and 1/2 of a green)
- 1/4 teaspoon salt
- 1/4 teaspoon ground black pepper
- 4 large eggs
- 1/3 cup shredded smoked gouda cheese

Optional:

- chopped fresh or dried parsley

Instructions

1. Begin shredding the potatoes by using the largest holes of your box grater. Wash and scrub the potatoes clean. You can peel them or leave the peels on, whichever you prefer. I always peel them when I make shredded hash. Place the shredded potato in a large bowl lined with a couple paper towels. Top with more paper towels and press down hard so the paper towels can absorb a lot of the moisture. You want a lot of the moisture gone, so just keep squeezing and using new paper towels as necessary. Alternatively, you can shred the potatoes onto a kitchen towel, wrap them up, and squeeze them out over the sink.

2. Transfer the shredded potatoes to a plate lined with two layers of paper towels. Cook in the microwave on high for 2 minutes– see notes in my post about why you are doing this. Set the potatoes aside.

3. Place a 10 – 12 inch skillet on the stove. Bacon should always begin in a cold pan, so before you turn the heat on, lay out your three strips on the pan. Then, turn the heat on low. Cook the bacon on both sides just before they become crispy. They will go back onto the stove and then in the oven, so they have more time to cook later in this recipe. Remove from heat, reserve the

grease, and set bacon on a plate lined with paper towels to absorb some grease. Once the bacon is slightly cool, you can chop it up.

4. Preheat oven to 400°F (204°C).

5. Turn the stove heat up to medium. When bacon grease begins to simmer, add the shredded potatoes. Give them a quick mix with a wooden spoon or rubber spatula. Allow to cook for about 2 minutes, untouched. Add the chopped pepper, salt, and pepper. Stir things around once or twice, then flatten everything out using the back of a wooden spoon or spatula. Allow to cook, untouched for 3 minutes. Stir, then allow to cook for 2 more minutes. The potatoes should be getting quite brown at this point. If not, continue to cook a little longer while stirring occasionally until they are. Stir in the chopped bacon and cook for 2 minutes. Remove skillet from the heat and flatten out the top of the hash using the back of a wooden spoon or spatula. Then, using the back of a spoon, make 4 shallow indentations into the hash. Crack an egg into each indentation. Top with shredded cheese (I usually sprinkle it around the eggs).

6. Transfer skillet to the oven and bake until the egg whites set, about 8-10 minutes. Season with salt and pepper to taste (usually I just add more pepper) and top with the parsley. Serve immediately.

Prep Time: 25 Minutes

Cook Time: 50 Minutes

Servings: 12

Ingredients

- 1 (12-14 ounce) loaf french bread, sourdough bread, or challah
- 1 cup (180g) fresh or frozen blueberries
- 8 large eggs
- 2 and 1/4 cups (540ml) whole milk
- 1/2 teaspoon ground cinnamon
- 3/4 cup (150g) packed light brown sugar
- 1 Tablespoon (15ml) pure vanilla extract
- Streusel Topping
- 1/3 cup (69g) packed light brown sugar
- 1/3 cup (41g) all-purpose flour (spoon & leveled)
- 1/2 teaspoon ground cinnamon
- 6 Tablespoons (86g) unsalted butter, cold and cubed

Optional:

- extra blueberries, fresh fruit, maple syrup, and/or confectioners' sugar for topping

Instructions

1. Grease a 9×13 inch pan with butter or spray with nonstick spray. Slice then cut the bread into cubes, about 1 inch in size. Spread cubes into the prepared baking pan and top evenly with blueberries. Set aside.
2. Whisk the eggs, milk, cinnamon, brown sugar, and vanilla together until no brown sugar lumps remain. Pour over the bread. Cover the pan tightly with plastic wrap and stick in the refrigerator for 3 hours – overnight. Overnight is best.
3. Preheat oven to 350°F (177°C). Remove pan from the refrigerator.
4. Prepare the topping: Whisk the brown sugar, flour, and cinnamon together in a medium bowl. Cut in the cubed butter with a pastry blender or two forks. Sprinkle the topping over the soaked bread.
5. Bake for 45-55 minutes or until golden brown on top. I usually bake it for 45 minutes because I like it softer. Serve immediately. Cover leftovers tightly and store in the refrigerator for 2-3 days.

11. Honey Garlic Soy Glazed Salmon

Prep Time: 15 Minutes

Cook Time: 20 Minutes

Servings: 4

Ingredients

- 4 salmon fillets, about 6 ounces (170g) each
- 1/3 cup (80ml) reduced sodium soy sauce (or regular)
- 1/3 cup (106g) honey
- 1 Tablespoon (15ml) sesame oil (or olive oil)
- 3 garlic cloves, minced (or 2 teaspoons jarred/minced)
- 1 teaspoon peeled minced fresh ginger

Optional:

- for garnish: chopped green onion and/or sesame seeds

Instructions

1. Marinate the salmon: Place salmon fillets into a large zippered food storage bag or shallow dish/container. In a medium bowl, whisk soy sauce, honey, sesame oil, garlic, and ginger together. Pour about half of the mixture (just eyeball it) over salmon. Turn salmon to coat. Seal the bag/cover the dish and refrigerate for at least 15 minutes and up to 4 hours.

2. Meanwhile, preheat oven to 375°F (191°C). Line a baking sheet with aluminum foil, parchment paper, or a silicone baking mat. Set aside.

3. Line the marinated salmon fillets on the baking sheet, skin side down. You can hold onto this used marinade—see step 5. Bake salmon for 15–20 minutes or until done, which is 10 minutes per inch thickness measured from the thickest part of the fillet. (Salmon is considered done when an instant read thermometer reads the center of the thickest part as at least 145°F (63°C).) Feel free to turn your oven to broil for the last minute to really crisp the edges.

4. Meanwhile, as the salmon bakes, pour the remaining unused marinade into a small saucepan or skillet over medium-high heat. If you want, you can add the remaining (used) marinade as well. Bring to a boil,

and then reduce heat to medium-low and simmer for 3–4 minutes or until slightly thickened. Keep a close eye on it because it can quickly burn. It will bubble up a lot as it reduces. Remove from heat.

5. Drizzle thickened glaze over baked salmon and serve with optional garnish.
6. Leftovers keep well in the refrigerator for a few days. Reheat to your liking.

Prep Time: 5 Minutes

Cook Time: 35 Minutes

Servings: 8

Ingredients

- 1 Tablespoon olive oil
- 3 garlic cloves, minced
- 1 cup chopped yellow onion (1/2 of a large onion)
- 1 Tablespoon Italian seasoning
- 3/4 teaspoon salt
- 3/4 teaspoon dried thyme
- 1/4 teaspoon fresh ground black pepper
- 8 cups beef, chicken, or vegetable broth
- 3–4 cups frozen, canned, or fresh vegetables
- 1 medium potato, peeled & chopped (1 heaping cup)
- 1 bay leaf
- 1 (6 ounce) can tomato paste
- 1 (14 ounce) can diced tomatoes (do not drain)
- 1 cup dry alphabet pasta

Instructions

1. Heat the olive oil over medium heat in a 5 quart (or larger) pot or dutch oven. Add the garlic, onion, Italian seasoning, salt, thyme, and pepper. Stir and cook for 5 minutes as the onion softens.

2. Add broth, vegetables, potato, bay leaf, tomato paste, and diced tomatoes. Bring to a boil, then add uncooked pasta. Cover and simmer for 30 minutes. Remove bay leaf.

3. Serve soup warm and top with fresh parmesan cheese, if desired.

4. Cover and store leftovers in the refrigerator for up to a week. To reheat, simply pour into a pot over medium heat and cook until warm. Feel free to add more broth to the leftovers as it cooks if it is too thick. (It thickens in the refrigerator as the potatoes and noodles soak up the liquid.)

Prep Time: 30 Minutes (add 3 hours for homemade dough)

Cook Time: 40 Minutes

Servings: 12

Ingredients

- 1 lb homemade rough puff pastry or store-bought frozen & thawed puff pastry (2 sheets)
- egg wash: 1 large egg beaten with 1 Tablespoon (15ml) water or milk

Topping:

- 1 Tablespoon (15ml) olive oil
- 2 cups (about 270g) peeled & sliced butternut squash (1/4 inch slices)
- 1 and 1/4 cups (150g) sliced or roughly chopped mushrooms
- 1/2 cup sliced onion (1/2 of a medium onion)
- 3 garlic cloves, minced
- 1/4 teaspoon salt
- pinch ground pepper, plus more for garnish
- 2 teaspoons fresh thyme leaves (or 1 teaspoon dried)

- 2 teaspoons chopped fresh rosemary (or 1 teaspoon dried)
- pinch ground nutmeg
- 1 cup (120g) shredded parmesan cheese

Optional for garnish:

- flaky sea salt, pepper, more cheese, more fresh thyme & rosemary

Instructions

1. Dough: Prepare homemade rough puff pastry dough through 2nd refrigeration. If using store-bought frozen puff pastry, make sure it's thawed. Keep either dough in the refrigerator until step 4 below.
2. Topping: Over low-medium heat in a large skillet, cook oil and butternut squash together for 5 minutes stirring occasionally. Add mushrooms, onion, garlic, salt, pepper, thyme, rosemary, and nutmeg. Cook until vegetables are soft, about 5-6 minutes. Remove from heat.
3. Preheat oven to 400°F (204°C). Line a large baking sheet with parchment paper or a silicone baking mat. Set aside.

4. On a lightly floured work surface using a lightly floured rolling pin, roll pastry dough into a 10×16 inch rectangle. (Tip if using store-bought– place the edge of one sheet over the other and use a rolling pin to adhere them together. Roll the whole thing out into a 10×16 inch rectangle.) Carefully transfer dough to lined baking sheet. If dough has lost shape, use your hands to reshape into a rectangle. Fold over a 1/2 inch edge and crimp edges down with a fork. Crimping is much easier the colder the pastry is, so place dough/baking sheet into the refrigerator to chill for 10 minutes if needed.

5. Egg Wash & Assemble: Brush egg wash all over puff pastry including the edges. Use a fork to poke holes all over the dough (not the crimped edge). Sprinkle with 3/4 cup (about 95g) cheese. Spoon vegetable topping over cheese and arrange in a single layer as best you can.

6. Bake tart for 30 minutes. Remove from the oven and sprinkle remaining cheese all over the top. Return to the oven and bake for 5-8 more minutes or until cheese is melted and pastry is golden brown.

7. Remove from the oven and, if desired, garnish with flaky sea salt, a sprinkle of pepper, and/or extra

cheese and herbs. Slice and serve warm or at room temperature.

Prep Time: 1hrs 5 Minutes

Cook Time: 20 Minutes

Servings: 2

Ingredients

Flatbread:

- 1 teaspoon active dry or instant yeast
- 1 teaspoon granulated sugar
- 3/4 cup (180ml) warm water, (between 100-110°F, 38-43°C)
- 2 cups (250g) all-purpose flour or bread flour (spoon & leveled), plus more for hands and surface
- 1 Tablespoon (15ml) olive oil, plus 1 teaspoon for brushing the dough
- 1 teaspoon salt

Toppings:

- 2 cups halved cherry tomatoes
- 1 Tablespoon + 1 teaspoon olive oil, divided
- salt & freshly ground black pepper
- 2 cups part-skim ricotta cheese

- 3 Tablespoons chopped fresh basil
- 2 Tablespoons milk, to thin
- 1–2 teaspoons fresh lemon juice
- 2 teaspoons minced garlic (or a few cloves, chopped)
- 2 cups sliced zucchini (about 1 medium/large)
- 6–8 ounces goat cheese (depending how much you like!)

Optional:

- crushed red pepper flakes and fresh basil to top

Instructions

1. Make the crust: Place the yeast and sugar in the bowl of a stand mixer fitted with a dough hook or paddle attachment. Or, if you do not own a stand mixer, a regular large mixing bowl. Pour warm water on top. Whisk gently to combine, then loosely cover with a clean kitchen towel and allow to sit for 5 minutes. The mixture should be frothy after 5 minutes. If not, start over with new yeast.

2. If you do not have a mixer, you can mix by hand in this step. With the stand mixer running on low speed, add the flour, olive, oil, and salt. Beat on low speed for 1 minute as it all combines. The dough should be thick and shaggy. Transfer it to a lightly floured work surface, including any loose flour. Knead it with lightly floured hands for 2 minutes until it begins to come together and becomes smooth. If the dough is too sticky to handle, add 1-2 more Tablespoons of flour.

3. Place the dough in a greased bowl (I use nonstick spray to grease) and cover with plastic wrap, aluminum foil, or a clean kitchen towel. Allow to sit and rest for 45 minutes at room temperature. Once it has rested and slightly risen, you can place it in the

fridge for up to 2 days. More instructions in the make ahead tip below.

4. As the dough is resting and rising, prepare the toppings. Toss the halved cherry tomatoes with 1 Tablespoon olive oil and a sprinkle of salt and pepper. Spread onto a parchment paper or silicone baking mat-lined baking sheet and bake in a 400°F (204°C) oven for about 20 minutes until blistered and roasted. Set aside.

5. Turn the oven up to 475°F (246°C).

6. Whisk the ricotta, basil, milk, lemon juice, and garlic together in a medium bowl. You can use a mixer for this if needed. Add salt and pepper to taste.

7. Shape the dough: Punch the dough down to release any air. Divide the dough into two. On a lightly floured surface with floured hands and working with one dough piece at a time, begin shaping and stretching the dough until it is 1/4 inch thick. You can use a floured rolling pin for this too. Don't worry about the shape of the dough, just make sure it's pretty thin. Repeat with the second piece of dough. Carefully transfer both pieces of dough to a parchment paper or silicone-mat lined baking sheet, or use a pizza stone. (You can also shape/roll out the

doughs directly on a silicone baking mat or a large sheet of parchment if that is easier for you and then just transfer the whole thing to the baking sheet.) Poke your fingers all around the surface of the flatbreads or prick a few holes with a fork. Drizzle or brush each with 1/2 teaspoon of olive oil.

8. Spread half of the ricotta mixture onto each, then top with zucchini, tomatoes, and finish them by crumbling the goat cheese on top of each.

9. Bake for 15-20 minutes or until the crust and toppings are browned to your liking. Remove from the oven and sprinkle with crushed red pepper, fresh basil, and/or freshly ground pepper. Slice and serve warm.

10. Cover and store leftovers in the refrigerator for up to 1 week.

Prep Time: 15 Minutes

Cook Time: 05 Minutes

Servings: 4

Ingredients

- 8 cups chopped romaine lettuce
- 1 pound strawberries, sliced
- 5–6 slices bacon, cooked and chopped
- 2/3 cup crumbled blue cheese
- 2/3 cup chopped pecans

Honey Balsamic Vinaigrette:

- 1/4 cup extra virgin olive oil
- 2 Tablespoons balsamic vinegar
- 2 Tablespoon honey
- 1 teaspoon dijon mustard
- Salt & freshly ground black pepper, to taste

Instructions

1. Make the vinaigrette first by whisking all of the vinaigrette ingredients together. Taste, then add salt and pepper as needed. You can make the dressing ahead of time and keep it in the refrigerator until ready to use. It's great for up to 2 weeks when stored in the refrigerator.

2. If your bacon is not already cooked, cook it according to its package directions. Cool until ready to handle, then chop it up.

3. In a large bowl, toss all of the salad ingredients together, then mix in the vinaigrette. You may not need all the vinaigrette– use as much or little as you prefer.

4. Plate and serve. Cover and store leftovers in the refrigerator for up to 2 days.

Prep Time: 15 Minutes

Cook Time: 05 Minutes

Servings: 4

Ingredients

Salad:

- 4 cups finely chopped kale (ribs removed)
- 2 cups cooked quinoa (about 2/3 cup dry)
- 3 medium blood oranges, peeled and chopped
- 1 avocado, peeled, cored and diced
- 5 oz blue cheese, crumbled
- 3/4 cup chopped walnuts

Blood Orange Vinaigrette:

- 1/3 cup olive oil
- 2 Tablespoons white wine vinegar
- 3 Tablespoons fresh blood orange juice
- 2 Tablespoons fresh lemon juice
- 1/4 teaspoon lemon zest
- 1 teaspoon honey

- 1/4 teaspoon sea salt

- freshly ground black pepper, to taste

Instructions

1. Combine all of the salad ingredients into a large bowl. Sometimes I do this with my hands to really mash up that avocado and massage it into the kale leaves.

2. For the dressing: Whisk all of the dressing ingredients together– or use a food processor. Pour dressing over salad and toss to coat everything evenly. Sometimes I don't use ALL the dressing– use however much you'd like. Store leftover dressing in the refrigerator for up to 2 weeks.

3. Serve immediately. Leftovers keep well in the refrigerator for 4-5 days.

Prep Time: 15 Minutes

Cook Time: 15 Minutes

Servings: 7-8

Ingredients

Creamy Greek Yogurt Buttermilk Dressing:

- 3/4 cup (180g) plain low fat Greek yogurt
- 1 cup (240ml) low fat buttermilk
- 2 Tablespoons low fat or regular mayonnaise
- 1 Tablespoon chopped fresh parsley
- 1 roasted garlic clove, minced
- 1 teaspoon white vinegar
- 1 teaspoon lemon juice
- 1/2 teaspoon salt
- 1/8 teaspoon ground black pepper

Pasta Salad:

- 1 pound dry pasta (we use fusilloni)
- 2 boneless skinless chicken breasts, grilled/cooked and chopped
- 1 pint cherry or grape tomatoes, halved

- 2 cups (350g) small broccoli florets
- 1 orange, green, yellow, or red bell pepper, chopped
- 1/2 cup (76g) crumbled feta cheese
- 3 strips crispy bacon, crumbled

Instructions

1. Make the dressing first: Whisk all of the dressing ingredients together. Taste, and add more salt/pepper/garlic/whatever you feel it needs. I usually add more roasted garlic and parsley. Stick the dressing in the refrigerator as you prepare the rest.

2. Make the pasta: Bring a large pot of salted water to a boil. Add the pasta and cook until al dente. Drain, then rinse with cold water to cool. Pour into a large bowl. Add the chicken, tomatoes, broccoli, and pepper. Pour 3/4 cup of the dressing over the pasta salad and gently toss to combine. Add a little more dressing if you'd like. Leftover dressing is great on salads – store in the fridge for up to 1 week.

3. Add the feta cheese and bacon and stir up the pasta salad again. Season with additional salt and pepper as desired. Chill for at least 2 hours and up to 1 day before serving to allow the flavors to settle. This

makes great leftovers! Cover tightly and store in the
refrigerator for up to 1 week.

Prep Time: 20 Minutes

Cook Time: 20 Minutes

Servings: 3

Ingredients

- 1 and 1/2 cups cooked quinoa
- 2 Tablespoons extra virgin olive oil
- 1 pound skinless boneless chicken breasts, cut into 1-inch pieces
- 2 cloves garlic or roasted garlic, finely chopped
- 1/2 teaspoon smoked paprika
- 1/2 teaspoon salt
- 2 large oranges, peeled and segmented
- 1 ripe avocado, sliced or cubed

Dressing

- 1/4 cup lime juice
- 1/3 cup chopped fresh cilantro (packed)
- 1 Tablespoon orange juice
- 1 Tablespoon extra virgin olive oil
- 1 Tablespoon honey

Instructions

1. Cook quinoa according to package directions. Transfer cooked quinoa to a large bowl and let cool.

2. Pour olive oil into a large skillet over medium heat. Add chicken and roasted garlic, stirring it all around to coat with oil. Sprinkle with smoked paprika and salt. Stir and cook until chicken is done, about 8 minutes. Add cooked chicken, oranges, and avocado to the quinoa. Stir to combine. Set aside.

3. Make the dressing: Whisk the dressing ingredients together. Pour over salad and toss to coat everything evenly. Serve immediately. Leftovers keep well in the refrigerator for 4-5 days.

Prep Time: 30 Minutes

Cook Time: 20 Minutes

Servings: 3-4

Ingredients

- 1 and 1/2 pounds skinless, boneless chicken breasts or tenders
- 1/2 cup whole wheat flour or all-purpose flour (spoon & leveled)
- 1 teaspoon salt
- 1/2 teaspoon ground black pepper
- 2 large eggs
- 1 and 1/2 cups finely crushed pretzels (or more, as needed)
- nonstick spray like PAM, olive oil spray, or coconut oil spray

Instructions

1. Preheat oven to 400°F (204°C). Line a large baking sheet with a silicone baking mat or coat heavily with nonstick spray.

2. If using chicken breasts, pound down and cut into little 1-1.5 inch pieces. If using boneless, skinless chicken tenders (chicken tenders are the lean strips of meat found attached to the underside of chicken breasts – they can also be purchased separately.) – simply cut into 1-1.5 inch pieces.

3. Combine flour, salt, and pepper in a shallow dish. Beat eggs in another shallow dish. Pour pretzels into a third shallow dish. Coat each chicken piece in flour, shaking off any excess. Then, dip in egg and let any excess drip off. Then generously roll in the pretzels, shaking off any excess. Add more crushed pretzels to the dish if you are running low. Place the chicken bites on the prepared baking sheet. Lightly spray each with nonstick spray to "seal" the breading, which will prevent the breading from staying raw and allows it to bake onto the chicken fingers.

4. Bake for 8 minutes. Turn each piece over and continue baking until the outside is crisp and the centers are cooked through, about 6-8 minutes more.

Baking times may vary, just make sure yours are cooked through. If you like them more brown, bake longer. Serve chicken bites with toothpicks (if using as an appetizer), honey mustard, or this spicy cheese sauce. Store any leftovers in the refrigerator for up to 2 days. I chopped them up and put on top of a salad. It was so good!

Prep Time: 30 Minutes

Cook Time: 20 Minutes

Servings: 3-4

Ingredients

- 1 and 1/2 pounds skinless, boneless chicken breasts or tenders
- 2 cups pecan halves
- 3 Tablespoons all-purpose flour (spoon & leveled)
- 1 teaspoon salt
- 1/2 teaspoon ground black pepper
- 1/2 teaspoon smoked paprika
- 2 large eggs
- chopped parsley for garnish, optional

Instructions

1. Set out 3 medium size bowls. Set aside. Preheat oven to 400°F (204°C). Line a large baking sheet with a silicone baking mat/parchment paper or coat heavily with nonstick spray. Set aside.

2. If using chicken breasts, pound down and cut into strips. If using boneless, skinless chicken tenders (chicken tenders are the lean strips of meat found attached to the underside of chicken breasts – they can also be purchased separately.) – cut in half lengthwise. Set aside.

3. Pulse 1/2 cup of pecan halves in a food processor or a blender until fine crumbs are formed. Be careful not to pulse into a nut butter, just a few pulses until they are ground up. See photo above in this post for a visual. In one of the medium bowls from step 1, mix the pecan crumbs with flour, salt, pepper, and paprika. Set aside.

4. Pulse the remaining pecan halves into coarse crumbs– larger pieces than the ground pecans from step 3. Pour them into another medium bowl. Finally, whisk the 2 eggs until beaten in the 3rd medium bowl.

5. Coat each chicken strip in the flour/ground pecan mixture, shaking off any excess. Then, dip in egg and let any excess drip off. Then, generously roll in the coarsely chopped pecans, shaking off any excess. Place the chicken strips on the prepared baking sheet.

6. Bake for 10 minutes. Turn each piece over and continue baking until the outside is crisp and the

centers are cooked through, about 10 minutes more. Baking times may vary, just make sure yours are cooked through. If you like them more brown, bake longer. Careful, you don't want to burn the nuts.

7. Serve chicken fingers with a garnish of parsley, some honey mustard, and/or your favorite condiment. Store any leftovers in the refrigerator for up to 2 days.

21. Homemade Flatbread Pizza

Prep Time: 55 Minutes

Cook Time: 15 Minutes

Servings: 2-4

Ingredients

- 1 teaspoon active dry or instant yeast
- 1 teaspoon granulated sugar
- 3/4 cup (180ml) warm water, (between 100-110°F, 38-43°C)
- 2 cups (250g) all-purpose flour or bread flour (spoon & leveled), plus more for hands and surface
- 1 Tablespoon (15ml) olive oil, plus 1 teaspoon for brushing the dough
- 1 teaspoon salt

Optional:

- 1 teaspoon garlic powder or 1 clove minced garlic and/or 1 teaspoon Italian seasoning

Instructions

1. Place the yeast and sugar in the bowl of a stand mixer
    fitted with a dough hook or paddle attachment. Or, if
    you do not own a stand mixer, a regular large mixing
    bowl. Pour warm water on top. Whisk gently to
    combine, then loosely cover with a clean kitchen towel
    and allow to sit for 5 minutes. The mixture should be
    frothy after 5 minutes. If not, start over with new
    yeast.

2. If you do not have a mixer, you can mix by hand in
    this step. With the stand mixer running on low speed,
    add the flour, olive oil, and salt. (And garlic/Italian
    seasoning if using.) Beat on low speed for 1 minute as
    it all combines. The dough should be thick and
    shaggy. Transfer it to a lightly floured work surface,
    including any loose flour. Knead it with lightly floured
    hands for 2 minutes until it begins to come together
    and becomes smooth. If the dough is too sticky to
    handle, add 1-2 more Tablespoons of flour.

3. Place the dough in a greased bowl (I use nonstick
    spray to grease) and cover with plastic wrap,
    aluminum foil, or a clean kitchen towel. Allow to sit
    and rest for 45 minutes at room temperature. Once it
    has rested and slightly risen, you can place it in the

fridge for up to 2 days. More instructions in the make ahead tip below.

4. As the dough is resting and rising, prepare your toppings. See blog post and/or recipe

5. Preheat oven to 475°F (246°C).

6. Shape the dough: Punch the dough down to release any air. Divide the dough into two. On a lightly floured surface with floured hands and working with one dough piece at a time, begin shaping and stretching the dough until it is 1/4 inch thick. You can use a floured rolling pin for this too. Don't worry about the shape of the dough, just make sure it's pretty thin. Repeat with the second piece of dough. Carefully transfer both pieces of dough to a parchment paper or silicone-mat lined baking sheet, or use a pizza stone. (You can also shape/roll out the doughs directly on a silicone baking mat or a large sheet of parchment if that is easier for you and then just transfer the whole thing to the baking sheet.)

7. Poke your fingers all around the surface of the flatbreads or prick a few holes with a fork. Drizzle or brush each with 1/2 teaspoon of olive oil. Top each with your favorite toppings.

8. Bake for 15-20 minutes or until the crust and toppings are browned to your liking. Remove from the oven. Slice and serve warm.

9. Cover and store leftovers in the refrigerator for up to 1 week.

Prep Time: 40 Minutes

Cook Time: 15 Minutes

Servings: 6

Ingredients

- 1 large egg
- 1/4 cup (60g) mayonnaise
- 1 Tablespoon chopped fresh parsley (or 2 teaspoons dried)
- 2 teaspoons dijon mustard
- 2 teaspoons worcestershire sauce
- 1 teaspoon Old Bay seasoning (up to 1 and 1/2 teaspoons for a spicier kick)
- 1 teaspoon fresh lemon juice, plus more for serving
- 1/8 teaspoon salt
- 1 pound fresh lump crab meat
- 2/3 cup (41g) Saltine cracker crumbs (about 14 crackers)

Optional:

- 2 Tablespoons (30g) melted salted or unsalted butter

Instructions

1. Whisk the egg, mayonnaise, parsley, dijon mustard, worcestershire sauce, Old Bay, lemon juice, and salt together in a large bowl. Place the crab meat on top, followed by the cracker crumbs. With a rubber spatula or large spoon, very gently and carefully fold together. You don't want to break up that crab meat!

2. Cover tightly and refrigerate for at least 30 minutes and up to 1 day.

3. Preheat oven to 450°F (232°C). Generously grease a rimmed baking sheet with butter or nonstick spray or line with a silicone baking mat.

4. Using a 1/2 cup measuring cup, portion the crab cake mixture into 6 mounds on the baking sheet. (Don't flatten!) Use your hands or a spoon to compact each individual mound so there aren't any lumps sticking out or falling apart. For extra flavor, brush each with melted butter. This is optional but recommended!

5. Bake for 12-14 minutes or until lightly browned around the edges and on top. Drizzle each with fresh lemon juice and serve warm.

6. Cover leftover crab cakes tightly and refrigerate for up to 5 days or freeze for up to 3 months.

Prep Time: 10 Minutes

Cook Time: 30 Minutes

Servings: 10-12

Ingredients

- 2 Tablespoons (30ml) olive oil
- 1 cup chopped yellow onion (1/2 of a large onion)
- 1 green bell pepper, diced
- 1 red bell pepper, diced
- 1 small jalapeño, minced (remove seeds and ribs)
- 3 garlic cloves, minced
- 1 teaspoon salt
- 1/2 teaspoon fresh ground black pepper
- 1/2 teaspoon ground cinnamon
- 2 and 1/2 teaspoons ground cumin
- 2 teaspoons chili powder
- 1 teaspoon onion powder
- 2 cups (480ml) vegetable broth
- 3 (14 ounce) cans petite diced tomatoes, do not drain
- 1 (15 ounce) can pinto beans, drained and rinsed
- 1 (15 ounce) can kidney beans, drained and rinsed

- 1 (15 ounce) can pumpkin puree
- 1 large sweet potato, peeled and diced (about 1 heaping cup)
- Optional: 1/2 (15 ounce) can black beans, drained and rinsed

Optional For Serving:

- cilantro
- Chopped red onion
- Sliced avocado

Instructions

1. Heat the olive oil over medium heat in a 5 quart (or larger) pot or dutch oven. Add the onion, bell peppers, and jalapeño. Stir and cook for 5 minutes as the onion softens. Add garlic, salt, black pepper, cumin, chili powder, and onion powder. Stir and cook for 1 minute. Add the remaining ingredients including black beans, if using.
2. Place the lid on top, reduce heat to medium-low, and cook for 30 minutes, stirring occasionally.
3. Serve with any optional toppings. I strongly suggest cilantro for a little fresh kick. Yum!

Prep Time: 2hrs 30 Minutes

Cook Time: 45 Minutes

Servings: 8

Ingredients

- 1 cup ricotta cheese, at room temperature
- 2 large eggs, at room temperature
- 3/4 cup shredded parmesan cheese (or other favorite cheese)
- 2 teaspoons minced garlic
- 1 Tablespoon favorite fresh herbs or 2 teaspoons dried herbs (I use a mix of thyme, rosemary, and parsley)
- 1/2 teaspoon salt
- pinch black pepper
- 1–2 cups thinly sliced vegetables such as sweet potatoes, zucchini, carrots, mushrooms, asparagus, brussels sprouts

Topping:

- 2 Tablespoons olive oil, coarse sea salt, more pepper + herbs

Instructions

The crust:

1. Prepare my pie crust recipe or butter pie crust through step 5.
2. After the pie crust has chilled, preheat the oven to 350°F (177°C).
3. Roll out the chilled pie dough and blind bake: On a floured work surface, roll out one of the discs of chilled dough (you can freeze the 2nd for later use, see note). Turn the dough about a quarter turn after every few rolls until you have a circle 12 inches in diameter. Carefully place the dough into a 9-inch tart pan.* Tuck it in with your fingers, making sure it is smooth. Fold the overhang edges back inward. See video above for a visual. Flute the edges of the crust. Chill for 20 minutes in the refrigerator or freezer. (Crust will shrink otherwise!) Line the chilled pie crust with parchment paper or aluminum foil. Fill with 2 sets of pie weights or dried beans. Bake for 15 minutes. Remove tart from the oven and carefully lift the parchment paper/aluminum foil (with the weights) out of the crust.

The filling:

1. Using a handheld or stand mixer fitted with a whisk attachment, beat the ricotta, eggs, parmesan cheese, garlic, herbs, salt, and pepper together until completely combined. Pour into warm crust. Arrange vegetable slices on top. Brush the vegetables and edges of the crust with olive oil , then sprinkle with sea salt, pepper, or more fresh herbs.

2. Bake for 30 minutes or until the vegetables and crust are lightly browned and crisp. After the first 15 minutes of bake time, place a pie crust shield on top of the tart to prevent the edges from browning too quickly. You can also tent a piece of aluminum foil over the whole tart if the top is browning too quickly.

3. Slice and serve tart warm or at room temperature. Cover and store leftover tart in the refrigerator for up to 1 week.

Freezing:

1. The baked and cooled tart freezes well for up to 3 months, tightly wrapped in a couple layers of plastic wrap or aluminum foil. Thaw overnight in the refrigerator and allow to come to room temperature before serving.

Prep Time: 2hrs 30 Minutes

Cook Time: 45 Minutes

Servings: 8

Ingredients

- 1 and 1/3 cups (320ml) warm water (between 100-110°F, 38-43°C)
- 2 and 1/4 teaspoons (7g) Platinum Yeast from Red Star instant yeast (1 standard packet)
- 1 Tablespoon (13g) granulated sugar
- 2 Tablespoons (30ml) olive oil, plus more for pan and brushing on dough
- 1 teaspoon salt
- 3 and 1/2 cups (about 450g) all-purpose flour (spoon & leveled), plus more for hands and surface
- Sprinkle of cornmeal for dusting the pan

Instructions

2. Whisk the warm water, yeast, and granulated sugar together in the bowl of your stand mixer fitted with a

dough hook or paddle attachment. Cover and allow to rest for 5 minutes. *If you don't have a stand mixer, simply use a large mixing bowl and mix the dough with a wooden spoon or rubber spatula in the next step.

3. Add the olive oil, salt, and flour. Beat on low speed for 2 minutes. Turn the dough out onto a lightly floured surface. With lightly floured hands, knead the dough for 3-4 minutes (for a visual, watch me do it in the video above!). The dough can be a little too heavy for a mixer to knead it, but you can certainly use the mixer on low speed instead. After kneading, the dough should still feel a little soft. Poke it with your finger – if it slowly bounces back, your dough is ready to rise. If not, keep kneading.

4. Lightly grease a large bowl with oil or nonstick spray– just use the same bowl you used for the dough. Place the dough in the bowl, turning it to coat all sides in the oil. Cover the bowl with aluminum foil, plastic wrap, or a clean kitchen towel. Allow the dough to rise at room temperature for 60-90 minutes or until double in size. (Tip: For the warm environment on a particularly cold day, heat your oven to 150°F (66°C). Turn the oven off, place the dough inside, and keep

the door slightly ajar. This will be a warm environment for your dough to rise. After about 30 minutes, close the oven door to trap the air inside with the rising dough. When it's doubled in size, remove from the oven.)

5. Preheat oven to 475°F (246°C). Allow it to heat for at least 15-20 minutes as you shape the pizza. (If using a pizza stone, place it in the oven to preheat as well.) Lightly grease baking sheet or pizza pan with nonstick spray or olive oil. Sprinkle lightly with cornmeal, which gives the crust extra crunch and flavor.

6. Shape the dough: When the dough is ready, punch it down to release any air bubbles. Divide the dough in half. (If not making 2 pizzas, freeze half of the dough for another time. See freezing instructions below.) On a lightly floured work surface using lightly floured hands or rolling pin, gently flatten the dough into a disc. Place on prepared pan and, using lightly floured hands, stretch and flatten the disc into a 12-inch circle, about 1/2-inch thick. If the dough keeps shrinking back as you try to stretch it, stop what you're doing, cover it lightly for 5-10 minutes, then try again. Once shaped into a 12-inch circle, lift the edge of the dough up to create a lip around the edges. I

simply pinch the edges up to create the rim. If using a pizza stone, place the dough directly on baker's peels dusted with cornmeal.

7. Cover dough lightly with plastic wrap or a clean kitchen towel and allow to rest for a few minutes as you prepare your pizza toppings. I suggest pepperoni & green peppers or jalapeño slices, extra cheese pizza, Hawaiian pizza, margherita pizza, pesto pizza, spinach artichoke white pizza, or homemade BBQ chicken pizza.

8. Top & bake the pizza: Using your fingers, push dents into the surface of the dough to prevent bubbling. To prevent the filling from making your pizza crust soggy, brush the top lightly with olive oil. Top with your favorite toppings and bake for 13-15 minutes or until the crust is golden brown.

9. Slice hot pizza and serve immediately. Cover leftover pizza tightly and store in the refrigerator. Reheat as you prefer. Baked pizza slices can be frozen up to 3 months.

Prep Time: 20 Minutes

Cook Time: 10 Minutes

Servings: 4

Ingredients

- 1 Tablespoon (15g) unsalted butter
- 2–3 cloves garlic, minced
- 2/3 cup (160ml) half-and-half, divided
- 1 lb medium or large uncooked shrimp, peeled & deveined
- 1 cup (about 200g) halved cherry tomatoes
- 1 Tablespoon (15ml) fresh lemon juice
- 1/2 cup (about 40g) parmesan cheese, freshly shredded
- 1 cup (240ml) store-bought or homemade pesto

Optional:

- fresh basil and extra parmesan cheese

Instructions

1. In a large skillet over medium heat, melt the butter.
   Add the minced garlic and 1/3 cup (80ml) half-and-
   half. Stir to combine, then bring the half-and-half to a
   simmer. Once simmering, add the shrimp. Cook for 1
   minute, then add the halved cherry tomatoes. Stir and
   cook until shrimp is nearly cooked through, just about
   pink on both sides. Stir in the remaining half-and-
   half, the lemon juice, and parmesan cheese. Cook for 1
   minute. (Shrimp should be fully cooked by this point.
   If not, keep cooking until it's pink.)

2. Remove from heat, then immediately stir in the pesto
   while everything is still hot. Serve plain, over cooked
   pasta, rice, or even zucchini noodles. Sprinkle with
   fresh basil and extra parmesan cheese, if desired.

3. Cover and store leftovers in the refrigerator for up to 5
   days.

Prep Time: 4hrs 20 Minutes

Cook Time: 10 Minutes

Servings: 4

Ingredients

- 4 large boneless skinless chicken breasts
- 1/3 cup (80ml) extra virgin olive oil, plus more for pan
- 1/4 cup (60g) dijon mustard
- 1/4 cup (60ml) dry white wine (or chicken broth)
- 3 garlic cloves, minced
- 1 teaspoon dried thyme
- 1 and 1/2 cups (190g) very finely chopped walnuts
- 1 cup (125g) all-purpose or whole wheat flour
- 1 teaspoon salt
- 1/2 teaspoon freshly ground black pepper

Optional:

- chopped fresh parsley for serving
- Honey Mustard Glaze
- 3 Tablespoons dijon mustard

- 1/3 cup (80g) honey

Instructions

1. Place the chicken, olive oil, mustard, white wine, garlic, and dried thyme in a large zipped-top bagger container. Seal shut, give it a shake to combine, and refrigerate for at least 4 hours and up to 12 hours.
2. Combine the walnuts, flour, salt, and pepper together in a shallow dish such as a 9×9 inch baking pan or a pie dish. Remove the chicken, shake off a little excess marinade and dip both sides of the chicken in the walnut mixture. Coat it really well so there's lots of walnut coating on each.
3. Preheat oven to 425°F (218°C).
4. Heat a couple Tablespoons of olive oil in an oven-safe skillet* over medium heat. Add the chicken and sear for 2 minutes, 1 minute on each side. Transfer skillet to the oven and bake, covered loosely with aluminum foil, for 15-20 minutes or until the chicken is fully cooked through. (Chicken is considered done when an instant read thermometer reads the center of the thickest part as at least 165°F (74°C).)

5. Whisk the glaze ingredients together and serve with chicken. Garnish chicken with fresh parsley if desired.

Prep Time: 20 Minutes

Cook Time: 10 Minutes

Servings: 10

Ingredients

Poppy Seed Dressing:

- 2/3 cup (160g) Greek yogurt
- 1/4 cup (60ml) apple cider vinegar
- 1/4 cup (60ml) extra virgin olive oil
- 1/4 cup (80g) honey
- 1/2 teaspoon salt
- 1/2 teaspoon ground dry mustard (or 1 teaspoon dijon mustard)
- 1 Tablespoon poppy seeds

Pasta Salad:

- 1 pound dry pasta (elbow, bow tie, rotini, etc)
- 5 cups chopped romaine lettuce
- 1 lb – 1.5 lbs strawberries, sliced (I use 1.5 lbs for lots of strawberries!)
- 2 avocados, diced

- 3/4 cup crumbled feta cheese
- 3/4 cup (85g) slivered or sliced almonds

Instructions

1. Cook pasta according to package directions. Drain and cool for 5 minutes.
2. Meanwhile, whisk all of the poppy seed dressing ingredients together.
3. Stir the remaining pasta salad ingredients in with the pasta. Toss with dressing. Add a little more feta and almonds if you wish. (I like a little extra cheese!)
4. Cover and store in the refrigerator for up to 1 week. Tastes best on day 2 or 3, so it's perfect to make ahead of time!

Prep Time: 20 Minutes

Cook Time: 30 Minutes

Servings: 8

Ingredients

- 1 pound (450g) dry elbow pasta or pasta shells
- 6 Tablespoons (86g) unsalted butter, divided
- 3 Tablespoons (24g) all-purpose flour
- 3 cups (720ml) whole milk
- 3 and 1/2 cups (about 14 ounces) shredded cheddar cheese
- 1/2 teaspoon each: salt, ground mustard, smoked paprika, and garlic powder
- dash of hot sauce (optional)
- 3 ounces (80g) brick-style cream cheese
- 1 cup (90g) Panko breadcrumbs

Optional for serving:

- finely chopped fresh parsley

Instructions

1. Preheat oven to 400°F (204°C).

2. In a large pot of boiling water, add a pinch of salt and the pasta. Cook the pasta until al dente, about 1-2 minutes less than the package cook time. Drain the cooked pasta, pour into a large bowl and stir in 2 Tablespoons of butter. Set pasta aside.

3. In a large saucepan or 12-inch oven-safe skillet, melt 2 Tablespoons of butter over medium heat. Once melted, whisk in the flour to form a thick paste. Cook and whisk the paste for 1 minute, then slowly whisk in the milk. Once all of the milk is added, continue to whisk. Bring to a simmer. Once simmering, whisk in the cheese until smooth. Whisk in the salt, ground mustard, smoked paprika, garlic powder, and hot sauce (if using). Cook for 2-3 minutes until thickened.

4. Pour the sauce over the buttered pasta. Add the cream cheese and stir everything together until the pasta is completely coated and cream cheese is melted. Scoop pasta back into skillet or a greased 9×13 inch pan.

5. Melt the remaining 2 Tablespoons of butter and mix with the Panko. Sprinkle over pasta.

6. Bake pasta for 30 minutes or until it is lightly browned on top and the sides are bubbling. I suggest

covering the pasta halfway through bake time to prevent the top from burning.

7. All to sit for 5 minutes before serving with a little fresh parsley. Careful, it's hot!

Prep Time: 20 Minutes

Cook Time: 8hrs 30 Minutes

Servings: 10-12

Ingredients

- 1 Tablespoon extra virgin olive oil
- 2 pounds 92-97% lean ground turkey (or beef)
- 4 Tablespoons taco seasoning, divided (2 standard packets or make your own!)
- 2 (14 ounce) cans petite diced tomatoes, drained
- 1 (7 or 8 ounce) can tomato sauce
- 2 cups chicken broth (we use reduced sodium)
- 1 large sweet potato, peeled and diced
- 1/2 cup yellow onion, diced
- 1 large green bell pepper, diced
- 1 (14 ounce) can corn (drained and rinsed) or 1 package of frozen corn
- 1 (14 ounce) can black beans, drained and rinsed
- 1 small jalapeño, minced (remove seeds and ribs)
- 1 Tablespoon ground cumin
- 1 teaspoon chili powder

- 1/2 teaspoon salt
- 1 hour before finishing: 1/2 cup uncooked & rinsed quinoa

Instructions

1. Heat oil in a large skillet over medium heat. Once hot, add the ground meat. Cook and stir for 4 minutes, then add 2 Tablespoons of taco seasoning. Stir and break up the meat as it cooks for another 4-5 more minutes, or until completely cooked through.
2. Transfer the cooked meat to a 5 quart or larger slow cooker. Add the remaining ingredients– including the remaining taco seasoning and except for the quinoa. Stir everything together until combined. Cook on low for 7 hours or on high for 4 hours.
3. Stir in the quinoa. Cook for 1 more hour on low or 30 more minutes on high.
4. Serve chili warm topped with chopped green onion, shredded cheese, sour cream, and/or avocado slices. Cover and store leftovers in the refrigerator for up to 1 week. Reheat in the microwave or on the stove.